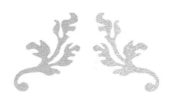

The Wood Pellet Grill Bible

A Survival Guide To Become A Pitmaster Of Your Wood Pellet
Grill With Delicious Bbq Recipes For Beginner And Advanced
Grillers To Impress Your Friends And Family

LIAM JONES

by any usage or abuse of any policies, processes, or Instructions contained within is the solitary and utter responsibility of the recipient reader. Under no circumstances will any legal responsibility or blame be held against the publisher for any reparation, damages, or monetary loss due to the information herein, either directly or indirectly.

The information herein is offered for informational purposes solely and is universal as such. The presentation of the information is without a contract or any type of guarantee assurance.

The trademarks that are used are without any consent and the publication of the trademark is without permission or backing by the trademark owner. All trademarks and brands within this book are for clarifying purposes only and are owned by the owners themselves, not affiliated with this document.

Table of Contents

BREAKFAST RECIPES 9

   1.   Cinnamon Sugar Pumpkin Seeds 10

   2.   Smoked Coconut 11

   3.   Blackberry Pie 13

   4.   S'mores Dip 15

FISH AND SEAFOOD RECIPES 18

   5.   Tuna Burgers 19

   6.   Grilled Clams with Garlic Butter 20

   7.   Simple but Delicious Fish Recipe 22

CHICKEN AND TURKEY RECIPES 24

   8.   Chicken Thighs with Salsa 24

   9.   Chicken Thigh Kebabs with Lime 27

   10.   Tasty Thai Chicken Satay 29

   11.   Crispy and Juicy Chicken 31

   12.   Glazed Chicken Thighs 33

   13.   Cajun Chicken Breasts 35

   14.   BBQ Sauce Smothered Chicken Breasts 36

   15.   Thanksgiving Dinner Turkey 38

BEEF RECIPES 41

16.   Baby Back Ribs 42

17.   Beef Jerky 44

18.   Beef Skewers 46

LAMB RECIPES 49

19.   Lamb Kebabs 49

20.   Ultimate Lamb Burgers 51

21.   Lamb Lollipops 53

22.   Lamb Chops 55

23.   Lamb Stew 57

PORK RECIPES 60

24.   Wood Pellet Grilled Pork Chops 60

25.   Wood Pellet Blackened Pork Chops 61

26.   Teriyaki Pineapple Pork Tenderloin Sliders 62

27.   Wood Pellet Togarashi Pork Tenderloin 64

APPETIZERS AND SIDES 66

28.   Garlic Parmesan Wedges 67

29.   Grilled Chili Lime Chicken 69

30.   Delicious Smoked Apple Pie 71

31.   Hearty Peaches 73

VEGETARIAN RECIPES 75

32. Corn Stuffed Zucchini...76

33. Wood Pellet Smoked Mushrooms........................77

34. Wood Pellet Grilled Asparagus and Honey Glazed Carrots 78

35. Wood Pellet Smoked Acorn Squash 80

GAME AND ORIGINAL RECIPES..............................83

36. Cinnamon Smoked Quails Orange Tea..............83

37. Roasted Venison Tenderloin...............................86

38. Grilled Game Hens with Rosemary sprig..........88

SNACKS...91

39. Empanadas...91

BREAKFAST RECIPES

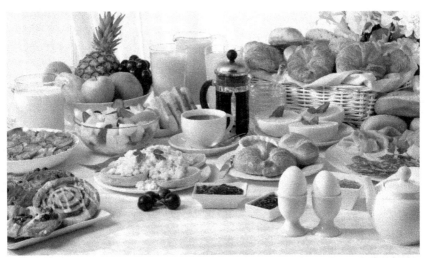

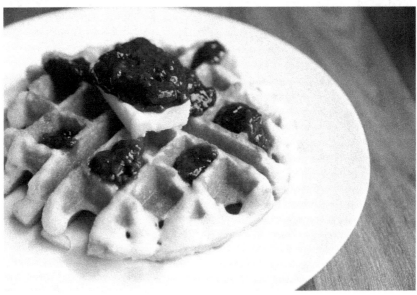

9

1. *Cinnamon Sugar Pumpkin Seeds*

Preparation Time: 15 minutes

Cooking Time: 30 minutes

Servings: 8

Ingredients:

- 2 tablespoons sugar
- Seeds from a pumpkin
- 1 teaspoon cinnamon
- 2 tablespoons melted butter

Directions:

1. Add wood pellets to your smoker and follow your cooker's startup procedure. Preheat your smoker, with your lid closed, until it reaches 350.

2. Clean the seeds and toss them in the melted butter. Add them to the sugar and cinnamon. Spread them out on a baking sheet, place them on the grill, and smoke for 25 minutes. Serve.

Nutrition: Calories: 127 Protein: 5g Carbs: 15g Fat: 21g

2. *Smoked Coconut*

Preparation Time: 10 minutes

Cooking Time: 30 Minutes

Servings: 4

Ingredients:

- 3 ½ cups flaked coconut
- 1 tbsp pure maple syrup
- 1 tbsp water
- 2 tbsp liquid smoke
- 1 tbsp soy sauce
- 1 tsp smoked paprika (optional)

Directions:

1. Preheat the smoker at 325°F.

2. Take a large mixing bowl and combine liquid smoke, maple syrup, soy sauce, and water.

3. Pour flaked coconut over the mixture. Add it to a cooking sheet.

4. Place in the middle rack of the smoker.

5. Smoke it for 30 minutes and every 7-8 minutes, keep flipping the sides.

6. Serve and enjoy.

Nutrition: Amount per 224 g = 1 serving(s) Energy (calories): 66 kcal Protein: 1.88 g Fat: 1.22 g Carbohydrates: 12.44 g

3. *Blackberry Pie*

Preparation Time: 15 minutes

Cooking Time: 40 minutes

Servings: 8

Ingredients:

- Butter, for greasing
- ½ cup all-purpose flour
- ½ cup milk
- 2 pints blackberries
- 2 cup sugar, divided
- 1 box refrigerated piecrusts
- 1 stick melted butter
- 1 stick of butter
- Vanilla ice cream

Directions:

1. Add wood pellets to your smoker and follow your cooker's startup procedure. Preheat your smoker, with your lid closed, until it reaches 375.
2. Butter a cast-iron skillet.
3. Unroll a piecrust and lay it in the bottom and up the sides of the skillet. Use a fork to poke holes in the crust.

4. Lay the skillet on the grill and smoke for five mins, or until the crust is browned. Set off the grill.

5. Mix 1 ½ c. of sugar, the flour, and the melted butter together. Add in the blackberries and toss everything together.

6. The berry mixture should be added to the skillet. The milk should be added to the top afterward. Sprinkle on half of the diced butter.

7. Unroll the second pie crust and lay it over the skillet. You can also slice it into strips and weave it on top to make it look like a lattice. Place the rest of the diced butter over the top. Sprinkle the rest of the sugar over the crust and place it skillet back on the grill.

8. Lower the lid and smoke for 15 to 20 minutes or until it is browned and bubbly. You may want to cover it with some foil to keep it from burning during the last few minutes of cooking. Serve the hot pie with some vanilla ice cream.

Nutrition: Calories: 393 Protein: 4.25g Carbs: 53.67g Fat: 18.75g

4. S'mores Dip

Preparation Time: 10 minutes

Cooking Time: 25 minutes

Servings: 8

Ingredients:

- 12 ounces semisweet chocolate chips
- ¼ cup milk
- 2 tablespoons melted salted butter
- 16 ounces marshmallows
- Apple wedges
- Graham crackers

Directions:

1. Add wood pellets to your smoker and follow your cooker's startup procedure. Preheat your smoker, with your lid closed, until it reaches 450.

2. Put a cast-iron skillet on your grill and add in the milk and melted butter. Stir together for a minute.

3. Once it has heated up, top with the chocolate chips, making sure it makes a single layer. Place the marshmallows on top, standing them on their end and covering the chocolate.

4. Cover, and let it smoke for five to seven minutes. The marshmallows should be toasted lightly.

5. Take the skillet off the heat and serve with apple wedges and graham crackers.

Nutrition: Calories: 216.7 Protein: 2.7g Carbs: 41g Fat: 4.7g

FISH AND SEAFOOD RECIPES

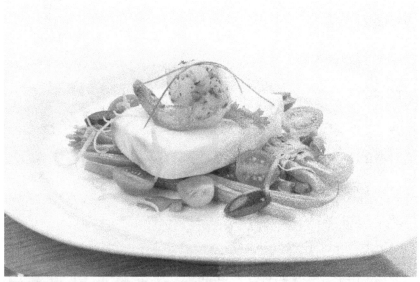

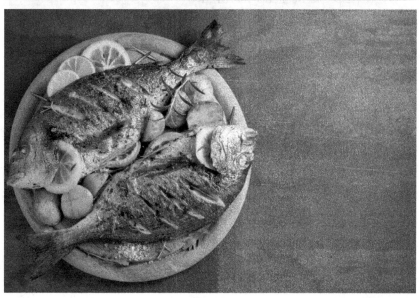

5. Tuna Burgers

Preparation Time: 30 minutes

Cooking Time: 15 minutes

Servings: 4-6

Pellet: Mesquite

Ingredients:

- 2 lbs. Tuna steak, ground
- 2 Eggs
- 1 Bell pepper, diced
- 1 tsp. Worcestershire or soy sauce
- 1 Onion, Diced
- 1 tbsp. Salmon rub seasoning
- 1 tbsp. Saskatchewan Seasoning

Directions:

1. A large bowl combines the salmon seasoning, Saskatchewan seasoning, bell pepper, onion, soy/Worcestershire sauce, eggs, and tuna. Mix well. Oil the hands and make patties.
2. Preheat the grill to high.
3. Grill the tuna patties for 10 - 15 min. Flip after 7 minutes.
4. Serve with topping you like and enjoy!

Nutrition: Amount per 228 g = 1 serving(s) Calories: 236 Protein: 18g Carbs: 1g Fat: 5g

6. *Grilled Clams with Garlic Butter*

Preparation Time: 10 minutes

Cooking Time: 8 minutes

Servings: 6-8

Pellet: Oak

Ingredients:

- 1 Lemon, cut wedges
- 1 - 2 tsp. Anise - flavored Liqueur
- 2 tbsp. Parsley, minced
- 2 - 3 Garlic cloves, minced
- 8 tbsp. butter, chunks
- 24 of Littleneck Clams

Directions:

1. Clean the clams with cold water. Discard those who are with broken shells or don't close.
2. Preheat the grill to 450F with a closed lid.
3. In a casserole dish, squeeze juice from 2 wedges, and add parsley, garlic, butter, and liqueur. Arrange the littleneck clams on the grate, grill for 8 minutes until open. Discard those that won't open.
4. Transfer the clams to the baking dish.
5. Serve in a shallow dish with lemon wedges. Enjoy!

Nutrition: Amount per 258 g = 1 serving(s) Calories: 273 Protein: 4g Carbs: 0.5g

Fat: 10g

7. *Simple but Delicious Fish Recipe*

Preparation Time: 45 minutes

Cooking Time: 10 minutes

Servings: 4-6

Pellet: Alder

Ingredients:

- 4 lbs. fish, cut it into pieces (portion size)
- 1 tbsp. minced Garlic
- 1/3 cup of Olive oil
- 1 cup of Soy Sauce
- Basil, chopped
- 2 Lemons, the juice

Directions:

1. Preheat the grill to 350°F with a closed lid.
2. Mix all the ingredients in a bowl. Then marinate the fish for 45 minutes.
3. Grill the fish until it reaches 145F internal temperature.
4. Serve with your favorite side dish and enjoy!

Nutrition: Amount per 380 g = 1 serving(s) Energy (calories): 730 kcal Protein: 59.07 g Fat: 48.26 g

Carbohydrates: 12.15 g

8. *Chicken Thighs with Salsa*

Preparation Time: 15 Minutes

Cooking Time: 10 Minutes

Servings: 8

Ingredients:

Marinade

- ¼ cup extra-virgin olive oil
- one orange, juiced
- half teaspoon ground cumin
- ¼ teaspoon ground coriander
- ¼ teaspoon cayenne pepper
- ¼ teaspoon smoked paprika
- one lime, juiced
- two cloves garlic, minced
- One pinch of salt and ground black pepper
- Eight thighs, bone, and skin removed skinless and boneless chicken thighs

Salsa

- One and a half cups diced and peeled fresh peaches

- One cup pitted and diced red cherries
- 1/3 cup chopped cilantro
- One tablespoon fresh lime juice
- Two tablespoons extra-virgin olive oil
- Two tablespoons seeded and minced jalapeno pepper
- Two tablespoons minced red onion

Directions:

1. Add lime juice, cumin, garlic, paprika, pepper, orange juice, olive oil, garlic, salt, coriander, lime juice, and cayenne to the bag. Close and squeeze the ingredients until it gets merged. Add chicken thighs and press out the excess air and then seal.

2. Place bag flat in the freezer so that chicken thighs are in one layer. Now, marinade for four hours and turn the bag over every two hours.

3. Set the salsa before the lighting grill. Mix cherries, cilantro, red onion, peaches, lime juice, and jalapeno in the bowl toss gently keep in the freezer

4. Now, clean and preheat the gas grill to the intermediate heat for twenty minutes.

5. Brush the grill grates utilizing olive oil and then remove the chicken thighs from the marinade.

6. Remove the marinade and grill chicken in one layer until it gets no longer pink in the middle for five to seven minutes on each side.

7. Take a thermometer and then insert it in the middle and it should read at least 165 degrees and then serve with salsa.

Nutrition: Calories 935 Total fat 53g Saturated fat 15g Protein 107g Sodium 320mg

9. *Chicken Thigh Kebabs with Lime*

Preparation Time: 20 Minutes

Cooking Time: 15 Minutes

Servings: 4

Ingredients:

Glaze:

- ¼ cup honey
- One tablespoon lime juice
- Two tablespoons Sriracha sauce

Kebabs:

- Eight large metal skewers
- One pound boneless and skinless chicken thighs
- Half small fresh pineapples
- one medium red onion,
- One red sweet pepper
- One medium zucchini
- two tablespoons olive oil
- one pinch of salt and freshly ground black pepper
- one pinch garlic powder,
- one teaspoon lime zest

Directions:

1. First, preheat the grill for intermediate to high heat and then lightly oil the grate.

2. Now, whisk lime juice, sriracha sauce, and honey in the little bowl and keep aside. Thread zucchini, red onion, pineapple, chicken, and red pepper on the skewers and put on the platter. Brush with olive oil and season with garlic powder, salt, and pepper.

3. Set skewers on the warm grate and seal lid and minimize the heat to intermediate. Grill until cooked completely and then turn the skewers for some minutes, at least fifteen to twenty minutes. Brush glaze on the skewers' whole sides for two to three minutes and then turn lightly caramelized glaze. Move to the serving plate and grate lime zest on the top and serve hot.

Nutrition: Calories 935 Total fat 53g Saturated fat 15g Protein 107g Sodium 320mg

10. _Tasty Thai Chicken Satay_

Preparation Time: 20 Minutes

Cooking Time: 10 Minutes

Servings: 8

Ingredients:

- Two tablespoons vegetable oil
- Two tablespoons soy sauce
- One teaspoon ground cumin
- One teaspoon ground coriander
- Two pounds skinless, boneless chicken breast
- Twenty wooden skewers
- Two tablespoons crunchy peanut butter
- Two tablespoons chopped peanuts
- One tablespoon lime juice
- One teaspoon muscovado sugar
- Two teaspoons tamarind paste
- One stalk lemongrass
- Two cloves garlic
- Half teaspoon chili powder
- One can of coconut milk
- Two teaspoons red Thai curry paste
- One tablespoon fish sauce

- One teaspoon tomato paste
- One tablespoon brown sugar

Directions:

1. Add lemongrass, soy sauce, tamarind paste, vegetable oil, garlic, muscovado sugar, cumin, chili powder, lime juice, and coriander in the blender to form a smooth paste. Take a plastic bag or a big bowl, toss chicken strips with marinade. Keep in the freezer for one hour.

2. Now, preheat the grill for intermediate to high heat and then lightly oil the grate.

3. Take a little saucepan and merge peanut, fish sauce, brown sugar, curry paste, peanut butter, coconut milk, and tomato paste. Cook it well and stir over the middle to low heat until it gets smooth and keeps hot.

4. Make a thread chicken on the skewers. Grill until it gets no longer pink in the middle for three to five minutes on every side. Serve with peanut sauce.

Nutrition: Calories 935 Total fat 53g Saturated fat 15g Protein 107g Sodium 320mg

11. *Crispy and Juicy Chicken*

Preparation Time: 15 Minutes

Cooking Time: 5 Hours

Servings: 6

Ingredients:

- ¾ C. dark brown sugar
- ½ C. ground espresso beans
- 1 tbsp. ground cumin
- 1 tbsp. ground cinnamon
- 1 tbsp. garlic powder
- 1 tbsp. cayenne pepper
- Salt and freshly ground black pepper
- 1 (4-lb.) whole chicken, neck, and giblets removed

Directions:

1. Set the temperature of the Wood Pellet Grill to 200-225 degrees F and preheat with a closed lid for 15 mins.
2. In a bowl, mix brown sugar, ground espresso, spices, salt, and black pepper.
3. Rub the chicken with spice mixture generously.
4. Put the chicken onto the grill and cook for about 3-5 hours.
5. Remove chicken from grill and place onto a cutting board for about 10 mins before carving.

6. With a sharp knife, cut the chicken into desired sized pieces and serve.

Nutrition: Calories per serving: 540 Carbohydrates: 20.7g Protein: 88.3g Fat: 9.6g Sugar: 18.1g Sodium: 226mg Fiber: 1.2g

12. Glazed Chicken Thighs

Preparation Time: 15 Minutes

Cooking Time: 30 Minutes

Servings: 4

Ingredients:

- 2 garlic cloves, minced
- ¼ C. honey
- 2 tbsp. soy sauce
- ¼ tsp. red pepper flakes, crushed
- 4 (5-oz.) skinless, boneless chicken thighs
- 2 tbsp. olive oil
- 2 tsp. sweet rub
- ¼ tsp. red chili powder
- Freshly ground black pepper, to taste

Directions:

1. Set the temperature of the Wood Pellet Grill to 400 degrees F and preheat with a closed lid for 15 mins.
2. In a small bowl, add garlic, honey, soy sauce, and red pepper flakes and with a wire whisk, beat until well combined.
3. Coat chicken thighs with oil and season with sweet rub, chili powder, and black pepper generously.

4. Arrange the chicken drumsticks onto the grill and cook for about 15 mins per side.

5. In the last 4-5 mins of cooking, coat the thighs with garlic mixture.

6. Serve immediately.

Nutrition: Calories per serving: 309 Carbohydrates: 18.7g Protein: 32.3g Fat: 12.1g Sugar: 17.6g Sodium: 504mg Fiber: 0.2g

13. Cajun Chicken Breasts

Preparation Time: 10 Minutes

Cooking Time: 6 Hours

Servings: 6

Ingredients:

- 2 lb. skinless, boneless chicken breasts
- 2 tbsp. Cajun seasoning
- 1 C. BBQ sauce

Directions:

1. Set the temperature of the Wood Pellet Grill to 225 degrees F and preheat with a closed lid for 15 mins.
2. Rub the chicken breasts with Cajun seasoning generously.
3. Put the chicken breasts onto the grill and cook for about 4-6 hours.
4. During the last hour of cooking, coat the breasts with BBQ sauce twice.
5. Serve hot.

Nutrition: Calories per serving: 252 Carbohydrates: 15.1g Protein: 33.8g Fat: 5.5g Sugar: 10.9g Sodium: 570mg Fiber: 0.3g

14. BBQ Sauce Smothered Chicken Breasts

Preparation Time: 15 Minutes

Cooking Time: 30 Minutes

Servings: 4

Ingredients:

- 1 tsp. garlic, crushed
- 2 tbsp. spicy BBQ sauce
- ¼ C. olive oil
- 1 tbsp. sweet mesquite seasoning
- 1 tbsp. Worcestershire sauce
- 4 chicken breasts
- 2 tbsp. regular BBQ sauce
- 2 tbsp. honey bourbon BBQ sauce

Directions:

1. Set the temperature of Wood pellet Grill to 450 degrees F and preheat with a closed lid for 15 mins.
2. In a large bowl, mix garlic, oil, Worcestershire sauce, and mesquite seasoning.
3. Brush chicken breasts with seasoning mixture evenly.
4. Place the chicken breasts onto the grill and cook for about 20-30 mins.
5. In the meantime, in a bowl, mix all 3 BBQ sauces.

6. In the last 4-5 mins of cooking, coat breast with BBQ sauce mixture.

7. Serve hot.

Nutrition: Calories per serving: 421 Carbohydrates: 10.1g Protein: 41.2g Fat: 23.3g Sugar: 6.9g Sodium: 763mg Fiber: 0.2g

15. _Thanksgiving Dinner Turkey_

Preparation Time: 15 Minutes

Cooking Time: 4 Hours

Servings: 16

Ingredients:

- ½ lb. butter, softened
- 2 tbsp. fresh thyme, chopped
- 2 tbsp. fresh rosemary, chopped
- 6 garlic cloves, crushed
- 1 (20-lb.) whole turkey, neck, and giblets removed
- Salt and freshly ground black pepper

Directions:

1. Set the temperature of Wood pellet Grill to 300 degrees F and preheat with a closed lid for 15 mins, using charcoal.
2. Place butter, fresh herbs, garlic, salt, and black pepper and mix well in a bowl.
3. With your fingers, separate the turkey skin from the breast to create a pocket.
4. Stuff the breast pocket with a ¼-inch thick layer of the butter mixture.
5. Season the turkey with salt and black pepper evenly.
6. Arrange the turkey onto the grill and cook for 3-4 hours.

7. Remove the turkey from the grill and place onto a cutting board for about 15-20 mins before carving.

8. With a sharp knife, cut the turkey into desired-sized pieces and serve.

Nutrition: Calories per serving: 965 Carbohydrates: 0.6g Protein: 106.5g Fat: 52g Sugar: 0g Sodium: 1916mg Fiber: 0.2g

BEEF RECIPES

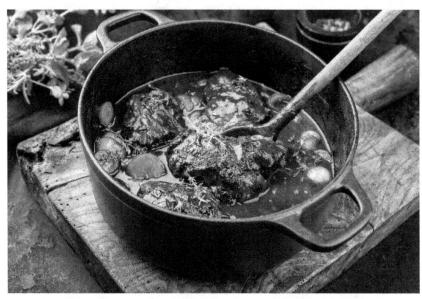

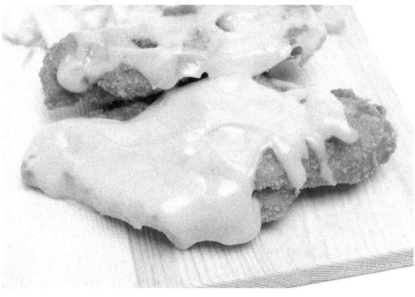

16. Baby Back Ribs

Preparation Time: 30 minutes

Cooking Time: 5 hours

Servings: 8

Ingredients:

- ½ cup BBQ sauce 1 rack baby back ribs
- 1 cup apple cider
- 1 tablespoon Worcestershire sauce
- 1 teaspoon paprika
- ½ cup packed dark brown sugar
- 2 tablespoon yellow mustard
- 2 tablespoon honey
- 2 tablespoon BBQ rub

Directions:

1. Remove the membrane on the back of the rib with a butter knife.
2. Combine the mustard, paprika, ½ cup apple cider, and Worcestershire sauce.
3. Rub the mixture over the rib and season the rib with BBQ rub.
4. Start your grill on the smoke setting and leave the lid open until the fire starts.

5. Close the lid and preheat the grill to 180°F using a hickory wood pellet.

6. Place the rib on the grill, smoke side up. Smoke for 3 hours.

7. Remove the ribs from the grill.

8. Tear off two large pieces of heavy-duty aluminum foil and place one on a large working surface. Place the rib on the foil, rib side up.

9. Sprinkle the sugar over the rib. Top it with honey and the remaining apple cider.

10. Place the other piece of foil over the rib and crimp the edges of the aluminum foil pieces together to form an airtight seal.

11. Place the sealed rib on the grill and cook for 2 hours.

12. After the cooking cycle, gently remove the foil from the rib and discard it.

13. Brush all sides of the baby's back rib with the BBQ sauce.

14. Return the rib to the grill grate directly and cook for an additional 30 minutes or until the sauce coating is firm and thick.

15. Remove the rib from the grill and let it cool for a few minutes.

16. Cut into sizes and serve.

Nutrition: Carbohydrates: 22g | Protein: 28g | Fat: 6g | Sodium: 13mg Cholesterol: 81mg

17. *Beef Jerky*

Preparation Time: 30 minutes

Cooking Time: 6 hours

Servings: 8

Ingredients:

- 1 cup pineapple juice
- ½ cup brown sugar
- 2 tablespoon sriracha
- 2 teaspoon onion powder
- 2 tablespoon minced garlic
- 2 tablespoon rice wine vinegar
- 2 tablespoon hoisin
- 1 teaspoon salt
- 1 tablespoon red pepper flakes
- 1 tablespoon coarsely ground black pepper
- 2 cups coconut aminos
- 2 jalapenos (thinly sliced)
- Meat:
- 3 pounds trimmed sirloin steak (sliced to ¼ inch thick)

Directions:

1. Combine all the marinade ingredients in a mixing bowl and mix until the ingredients are well combined.

2. Put the sliced sirloin in a gallon-sized zip-lock bag and pour the marinade into the bag. Massage the marinade into the beef. Seal the bag and refrigerate for 8 hours.

3. Remove the zip-lock bag from the refrigerator.

4. Activate the pellet grill smoker setting and leave the lip opened for 5 minutes until the fire starts.

5. Close the lid and preheat your pellet grill to 180°F, using a hickory pellet.

6. Remove the beef slices from the marinade and pat them dry with a paper towel.

7. Arrange the beef slice on the grill in a single layer. Smoke the beef for about 4 to 5 hours, turning often after the first 2 hours of smoking. The jerky should be dark and dry when it is done.

8. Remove the jerky from the grill and let it sit for about 1 hour to cool.

9. Serve immediately or store in an airtight container and refrigerate for future use.

Nutrition: Carbohydrates: 12g | Protein: 28g | Fat: 16g | Sodium: 23mg Cholesterol: 21mg

18. Beef Skewers

Preparation Time: 30 minutes

Cooking Time: 5 hours

Servings: 8

Ingredients:

- 2 tablespoon olive oil
- 2 pounds top round steak (cut to ¼-inch-thick and 2-inch-wide slices)
- 2 garlic cloves (finely chopped)
- ¼ cup water
- ½ cup soy sauce
- ¾ cup brown sugar
- 1 tablespoon minced fresh ginger
- 1 teaspoon freshly ground black pepper or more to taste
- 3 tablespoon red wine vinegar
- 3 tablespoon dried basil
- Wooden or bamboo skewers (soaked in water for 30 minutes, at least)

Directions:

1. In a mixing bowl, combine the olive oil, sugar, ginger, garlic, soy sauce, water, vinegar, pepper, and basil. Mix until the ingredients are well combined.

2. Pour the marinade into a zip-lock bag and add the steak slices. Massage the marinade into the steak slices. Refrigerate for 12 hours or more.

3. Remove the steak slices from the marinade and pat them dry with a paper towel.

4. Thread the steak slices onto the soaked skewers.

5. Activate the smoke setting on your wood smoker grill, using a hickory wood pellet. Leave the lid open until the fire is established.

6. Close the lid and preheat the grill to 325°F for direct-heat cooking.

7. Arrange the skewered steak onto the grill and grill for 8 minutes or until the meat is done, turning occasionally.

8. Remove the skewered meat from the grill and let them sit for a few minutes to cool.

9. Serve warm and enjoy.

Nutrition: Carbohydrates: 12g | Protein: 28g | Fat: 16g | Sodium: 23mg Cholesterol: 21mg

19. *Lamb Kebabs*

Preparation Time: 15 minutes

Cooking Time: 10 minutes

Servings: 4

Ingredients

- 1/2 tablespoon salt
- 2 tablespoons fresh mint
- 3 lbs. leg of lamb
- 1/2 cup lemon juice
- 1 tablespoon lemon zest
- 15 apricots, pitted
- 1/2 tablespoon cilantro
- 2 teaspoons black pepper
- 1/2 cup olive oil
- 1 teaspoon cumin
- 2 red onion

Directions:

1. In a bowl, mix the olive oil, pepper, lemon juice, mint, salt, lemon zest, cumin, and cilantro. Add lamb leg, then place in the refrigerator overnight.

2. Remove the lamb from the marinade, cube them, and then thread onto the skewer with the apricots and onions.

3. When ready to cook, turn your smoker to 400 deg and preheat.

4. Lay the skewers on the grill and cook for ten minutes.

5. Remove from the grill and serve.

Nutrition: Calories 390, Total fat 35g, Saturated fat 15g, Total Carbs 0g, Net Carbs 0g, Protein 17g, Sugar 0g, Fiber 0g, Sodium: 65mg.

20. Ultimate Lamb Burgers

Preparation Time: 20 minutes

Cooking Time: 30 minutes

Servings: 4

Ingredients

- Burger:
- 2 lbs. ground lamb
- 1 jalapeño
- 6 scallions, diced
- 2 tablespoons mint
- 2 tablespoons dill, minced
- 3 cloves garlic, minced
- Salt and pepper
- 4 brioche buns
- 4 slices manchego cheese
- Sauce:
- 1 cup mayonnaise
- 2 teaspoons lemon juice
- 2 cloves garlic
- 1 bell pepper, diced
- salt and pepper

Directions:

1. When ready to cook, turn your smoker to 400 deg and preheat.

2. Add the mint, scallions, salt, garlic, dill, jalapeño, lamb, and pepper to the mixing bowl.

3. Form the lamb mixture into eight patties.

4. Lay the pepper on the grill and cook for 20 minutes.

5. Take the pepper from the grill and place it in a bag, and seal. After ten minutes, remove pepper from the bag, remove seeds and peel the skin.

6. Add the garlic, lemon juice, mayo, roasted red pepper, salt, and pepper, and process until smooth. Serve alongside the burger.

7. Lay the lamb burgers on the grill, and cook for five minutes per side, then place in the buns with a slice of cheese, and serve with the homemade sauce.

Nutrition: Calories 390, Total fat 35g, Saturated fat 15g, Total Carbs 0g, Net Carbs 0g, Protein 17g, Sugar 0g, Fiber 0g, Sodium: 65mg.

21. Lamb Lollipops

Preparation Time: 15 minutes

Cooking Time: 10 minutes

Servings: 4

Ingredients

- 6 lamb chops
- 2 tablespoons olive oil
- 1/2 tablespoon salt
- Chutney:
- 1 mango
- 3 cloves garlic
- 1/2 habanero pepper
- 3 sprigs cilantro
- 1 tablespoon lime juice
- 1 teaspoon salt
- 5 tablespoons pepper
- 2 tablespoons mint

Directions:

1. Start by cutting the fat off your lamb chops.
2. Mix all of the chutney ingredients in a processor until well blended and smooth.

3. When ready to cook, turn your smoker to 400 deg and preheat.

4. Drizzle the lamb with olive oil and season with salt and pepper before grilling for five minutes on each side, then leave to rest.

5. Serve with chutney and chopped mint.

Nutrition: Calories 390, Total fat 35g, Saturated fat 15g, Total Carbs 0g, Net Carbs 0g, Protein 17g, Sugar 0g, Fiber 0g, Sodium: 65mg.

22. *Lamb Chops*

Preparation Time: 15 minutes

Cooking Time: 15 minutes

Servings: 4

Ingredients

- 1/2 cup extra-virgin olive oil
- 1/4 cup onion, diced
- 2 cloves garlic, minced
- 2 tablespoons soy sauce
- 2 tablespoons balsamic vinegar
- 1 tablespoon rosemary
- 2 teaspoons mustard
- 1 teaspoon Worcestershire sauce
- 8 oz. lamb chops
- Salt and pepper

Directions:

1. In a pan, sauté the onion with garlic and olive oil over medium heat.
2. Take the mixture and place it in a blender with vinegar, soy sauce, rosemary, Worcestershire sauce, and mustard.
3. Next, season the mixture with black pepper and set it to one side.

4. When ready to cook, set the smoker temperature to 500 deg and preheat.

5. Brush the lamb chops with olive oil and season with salt and pepper.

6. Smoke the lamb chops for six minutes per side. Serve alongside your homemade sauce.

Nutrition: Calories 390, Total fat 35g, Saturated fat 15g, Total Carbs 0g, Net Carbs 0g, Protein 17g, Sugar 0g, Fiber 0g, Sodium: 65mg.

23. Lamb Stew

Preparation Time: 45 minutes

Cooking Time: 1 hour

Servings: 4

Ingredients

- 2 tablespoons olive oil
- 3 lbs. lamb
- 4 cloves garlic
- 1/4 cup tomato paste
- 2 cups beef stock
- 2 tablespoons dried thyme
- 2 bay leaves
- Salt and pepper
- 12 oz. stout beer
- 3 carrots, peeled and diced
- 1 turnip, peeled and chopped
- 2 onions, chopped
- 1 large parsnip, peeled and chopped
- 2 potatoes, chopped

Directions:

1. When ready to cook, set your smoker to 450 deg and preheat.
2. Season your lamb with salt and pepper.

3. Dice the lamb and cook in the smoker in a large pot, eight minutes on each side, before adding garlic, beef stock, thyme, beer, bay leaves, and salt to the mix and cooking for ten minutes.

4. Add the remaining vegetables and cook for another 50 minutes before serving.

Nutrition: Calories 390, Total fat 35g, Saturated fat 15g, Total Carbs 0g, Net Carbs 0g, Protein 17g, Sugar 0g, Fiber 0g, Sodium: 65mg.

PORK RECIPES

24. *Wood Pellet Grilled Pork Chops*

Preparation Time: 20 Minutes

Cooking Time: 10 Minutes

Servings: 6

Ingredients:

- Six pork chops, thickly cut
- BBQ rub

Directions:

1. Preheat the wood pellet to 450°F.
2. Season the pork chops generously with the BBQ rub. Place the pork chops on the grill and cook for 6 minutes or until the internal temperature reaches 145°F.
3. Remove from the grill and let sit for 10 minutes before serving.
4. Enjoy.

Nutrition: Calories 264 Total fat 13g Saturated fat 6g Total Carbs 4g Net Carbs 1g Protein 33g Fiber 3g Sodium: 66mg

25. Wood Pellet Blackened Pork Chops

Preparation Time: 5 Minutes

Cooking Time: 20 Minutes

Servings: 6

Ingredients:

- Six pork chops
- 1/4 cup blackening seasoning
- Salt and pepper to taste

Directions:

1. Preheat your grill to 375°F.
2. Meanwhile, generously season the pork chops with the blackening seasoning, salt, and pepper.
3. Place the pork chops on the grill and close the lid.
4. Let grill for 8 minutes, then flip the chops. Cook until the internal temperature reaches 142°F.
5. Remove the chops from the grill and let rest for 10 minutes before slicing.
6. Serve and enjoy.

Nutrition: Calories 333 Total fat 18g Saturated fat 6g Total Carbs 1g Protein 40g, Fiber 1g Sodium: 3175mg

26. Teriyaki Pineapple Pork Tenderloin Sliders

Preparation Time: 20 Minutes

Cooking Time: 20 Minutes

Servings: 6

Ingredients:

- 1-1/2 lb. pork tenderloin
- One can pineapple ring
- One package king's Hawaiian rolls
- 8 oz teriyaki sauce
- 1-1/2 tbsp salt
- 1 tbsp onion powder
- 1 tbsp paprika
- 1/2 tbsp garlic powder
- 1/2 tbsp cayenne pepper

Directions:

1. Add all the fixings for the rub in a mixing bowl and mix until well mixed. Generously rub the pork loin with the mixture.
2. Heat the pellet to 325°F. Place the meat on a grill and cook while you turn it in every 4 minutes.
3. Cook until the internal temperature reaches 145°F.remove from the grill and let it rest for 5 minutes.

4. Meanwhile, open the pineapple can and place the pineapple rings on the grill. Flip the crews when they have a dark brown color.

5. At the same time, half the rolls and place them on the grill and grill them until toasty browned.

6. Assemble the slider by putting the bottom roll first, followed by the pork tenderloin, pineapple ring, a drizzle of sauce, and top with the other roll half. Serve and enjoy.

Nutrition: Calories 243 Total fat 5g Saturated fat 2g Total Carbs 4g Net Carbs 15g Protein 33g Sugar 10g, Fiber 1g Sodium: 2447mg

27. *Wood Pellet Togarashi Pork Tenderloin*

Preparation Time: 5 Minutes

Cooking Time: 25 Minutes

Servings: 6

Ingredients:

- 1 Pork tenderloin
- 1/2tbsp kosher salt
- 1/4 cup Togarashi seasoning

Directions:

1. Cut any excess silver skin from the pork and sprinkle with salt to taste. Rub generously with the togarashi seasoning
2. Place in a preheated oven at 400°F for 25 minutes or until the internal temperature reaches 145°F.
3. Remove from the grill and let rest for 10 minutes before slicing and serving.
4. Enjoy.

Nutrition: Calories 390 Total fat 13g Saturated fat 6g Total Carbs 4g Net Carbs 1g Protein 33g Sugar 0g Fiber 3g Sodium: 66mg

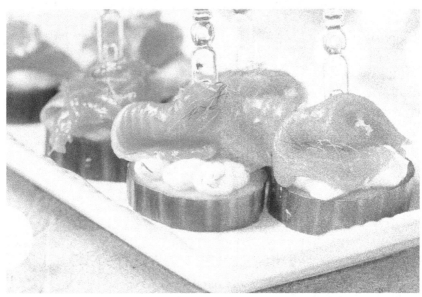

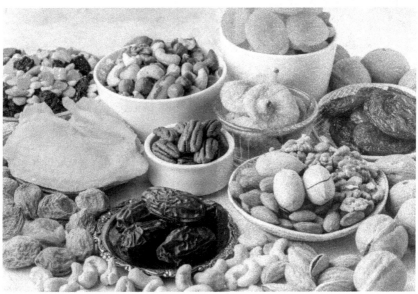

28. Garlic Parmesan Wedges

Preparation Time: 15 min

Cooking Time: 35 min

Servings: 3

Ingredients:

- 3 russet potatoes (large)
- 2 teaspoons of garlic powder
- ¾ teaspoon black pepper
- 1 ½ teaspoon of salt
- ¾ cup Parmesan cheese (grated)
- 3 tablespoons fresh cilantro (chopped, optional. You can replace this with flat-leaf parsley)
- ½ cup blue cheese (per serving, as an optional dip. Can be replaced with ranch dressing)

Directions:

1. Use some cold water to scrub your potatoes as gently as you can with a veggie brush. When done, let them dry.
2. Slice your potatoes along the length in half. Cut each half into a third.
3. Get all the extra moisture off your potato by wiping it all away with a paper towel. If you don't do this, then you're not going to have crispy wedges!

4. In a large bowl, throw in your potato wedges, some olive oil, garlic powder, salt, garlic, and pepper, and then toss them with your hands, lightly. You want to make sure the spices and oil get on every wedge.

5. Place your wedges on a nonstick grilling tray, or pan, or basked. The single-layer kind. Make sure it's at least 15 x 12 inches.

6. Set up your wood pellet smoker grill so it's ready for indirect cooking.

7. Preheat your grill to 425°F, with whatever wood pellets you like.

8. Set the grilling tray upon your preheated grill. Roast the wedges for 15 minutes before you flip them. Once you turn them, roast them for another 15 minutes, or 20 tops. The outside should be a nice, crispy, golden brown.

9. Sprinkle your wedges generously with the Parmesan cheese. When you're done, garnish it with some parsley, or cilantro, if you like. Serve these bad boys up with some ranch dressing, or some blue cheese, or just eat them that way!

Nutrition: Calories: 194 Fat: 5g Cholesterol: 5mg Carbs: 32g Protein: 5g Intolerances: Gluten-Free, Egg-Free

29. *Grilled Chili Lime Chicken*

Preparation Time:10 MIN

Cooking Time:10 MIN

Servings:4

Ingredients

- ¼ cup fresh lime juice

- One lime, zested

- One teaspoon red pepper flakes

- Half teaspoon ground cumin

- One teaspoon salt

- One teaspoon brown sugar

- Four medium skinless, boneless chicken breast halves

- Two tablespoons chopped fresh cilantro

- Two tablespoons olive oil

- Two cloves garlic, minced

Directions:

1. First, take a little bowl and whisk lime juice, lime zest, cumin, olive oil, brown sugar, garlic, salt, and red pepper flakes. Add chicken to the bowl or big plastic bag and then add the lime marinade. Seal the bag and wrap the bowl and keep it in the freezer to preserve for a half-hour to one day.

2. Now, preheat the grill middle to high heat and lightly oil the grate.
3. Add chicken breasts on the preheated grill and fry until it gets white in the middle and the skin gets golden and lightly charred. Cook approx. five minutes per side.
4. Move chicken breast to the plate and allow stand for five minutes and cut and decorate with cilantro.

Nutrition: Calories: 194 Fat: 5g Cholesterol: 5mg Carbs: 32g Protein: 5g Intolerances: Gluten-Free, Egg-Free

30. *Delicious Smoked Apple Pie*

Preparation Time: 10-15 minutes

Cooking Time: 20-30 minutes

Servings; 4

Ingredients

- 5 apples
- ¼ cup of sugar
- 1 tablespoon cornstarch
- Flour as needed
- 1 refrigerated pie crust
- ¼ cup peach preserve

Directions:

1. Take your drip pan and add water, cover with aluminum foil. Pre-heat your smoker to 275 degrees F
2. Use water fill water pan halfway through and place it over drip pan. Add wood chips to the side tray
3. Take a medium-sized bowl and add apples, sugar, cornstarch and stir well until combined thoroughly
4. Transfer to one side
5. Dust a work surface with flour and roll out your pie crust
6. Transfer pie crust into a pie pan (no greasing)
7. Spread preserve on bottom of pan and top with apple slices

8. Transfer into smoker and smoke for 30-40 minutes

9. Serve and enjoy!

Nutrition; Calories: 236 Fat: 9g Carbohydrates: 39g Protein: 2g

31. Hearty Peaches

Preparation Time: 10-15 minutes

Cooking Time: 30 minutes

Servings: 4

Ingredients

- 6 fresh peaches

Directions:

1. Take your drip pan and add water, cover with aluminum foil. Pre-heat your smoker to 200 degrees F

2. Use water fill water pan halfway through and place it over drip pan. Add wood chips to the side tray

3. Transfer peaches directly onto your smoker and smoke for 30 minutes, the first 20 minutes should be skin side down while the final 10 should be skin side up

4. Remove from smoker and serve, enjoy!

Nutrition; Calories: 117 Fat: 0.8g Carbohydrates: 28g Protein: 3g

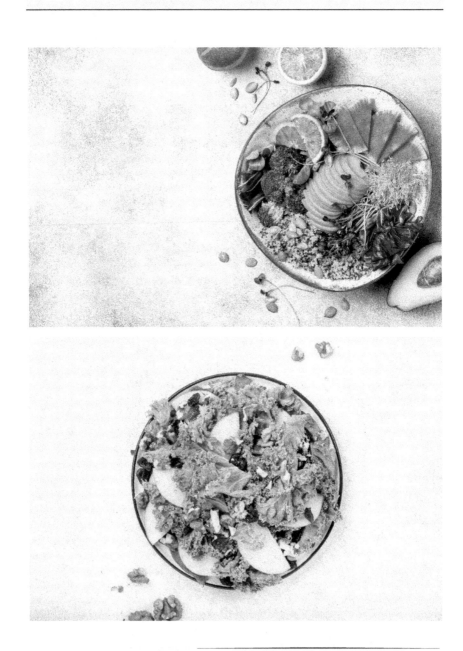

32. Corn Stuffed Zucchini

Preparation Time: 15 minutes

Cooking Time: 40 minutes

Servings: 3

Ingredients:

- 3 medium Zucchini (cut in half lengthwise)
- 1 egg
- 1/2 cup feta cheese (crumbled)
- 1/3 cup shredded cheddar cheese
- 1 can corn
- 1/2 tsp salt
- 1/2 tsp ground black pepper

Directions:

1. Preheat the Electric Smoker to 275F. Scoop out the Zucchini seeds and some pulp into a bowl, add the feta cheese, corn, egg, cheddar cheese, salt, pepper, and mix. Spoon the mixture into the hollowed zucchini.
2. Transfer the stuffed zucchinis into the smoker and smoke for 30 minutes, top with more cheese, and smoke for an additional 10 minutes or until the cheese is melted. Serve.

Nutrition: Calories: 121 Carbs: 14g Fat: 6g Protein: 13.2g

33. *Wood Pellet Smoked Mushrooms*

Preparation Time: 15 minutes,

Cooking Time: 45 minutes.

Servings: 5

Ingredients:

- 4 cup Portobello, whole and cleaned
- 1 tbsp. canola oil
- 1 tbsp. onion powder
- 1 tbsp. granulated garlic
- 1 tbsp. salt
- 1 tbsp. pepper

Directions:

1. Put all the ingredients and mix well.
2. Set the wood pellet temperature to 180°F then place the mushrooms directly on the grill.
3. Smoke the mushrooms for 30 minutes.
4. Increase the temperature to high and cook the mushrooms for a further 15 minutes.
5. Serve and enjoy.

Nutrition: Calories: 1680 Fat: 30g Carbs: 10g Protein: 4g Sodium: 514mg, Potassium: 0mg:

34. Wood Pellet Grilled Asparagus and Honey Glazed Carrots

Preparation Time: 15 minutes

Cooking Time: 35 minutes

Servings: 5

Ingredients:

- 1 bunch asparagus, trimmed ends
- 1 lb. carrots, peeled
- 2 tbsp. olive oil
- Sea salt to taste
- 2 tbsp. honey
- Lemon zest

Directions:

1. Sprinkle the asparagus with oil and sea salt. Drizzle the carrots with honey and salt.

2. Preheat the wood pellet to 165°F with the lid closed for 15 minutes.

3. Place the carrots in the wood pellet and cook for 15 minutes. Add asparagus and cook for 20 more minutes or until cooked through.

4. Top the carrots and asparagus with lemon zest. Enjoy.

Nutrition: Calories: 1680 Total Fat: 30g Saturated Fat: 2g Total Carbs: 10g Net Carbs: 10g Protein: 4g Sodium: 514mg

35. *Wood Pellet Smoked Acorn Squash*

Preparation Time: 10 minutes

Cooking Time: 2 hours

Servings: 6

Ingredients:

- 3 tbsp. olive oil
- 3 acorn squash, halved and seeded
- 1/4 cup unsalted butter
- 1/4 cup brown sugar:
- 1 tbsp. cinnamon, ground
- 1 tbsp. chili powder
- 1 tbsp. nutmeg, ground

Directions:

1. Brush olive oil on the acorn squash cut sides then cover the halves with foil. Poke holes on the foil to allow steam and smoke through.
2. Fire up the wood pellet to 225°F and smoke the squash for 1 ½-2 hour.
3. Remove the squash from the smoker and allow it to sit.
4. Meanwhile, melt butter, Sugar: and spices in a saucepan. Stir well to combine.

5. Remove the foil from the squash and spoon the butter mixture in each squash half. Enjoy.

Nutrition: Calories: 149 Total Fat: 10g Saturated Fat: 5g Total Carbs: 14g Net Carbs: 12g

Protein: 2g Sugar: 0g Fiber: 2g Sodium: 19mg Potassium: 0mg

36. *Cinnamon Smoked Quails Orange Tea*

Preparation Time: 10 minutes

Cooking Time: 1 hour 10 minutes

Servings: 10

Ingredients:

- Quails (6-lb., 2.7-kg.)
- The Rub:
- ¼ cup Sichuan peppercorns
- 2 tbsp. Kosher salt
- 1 tsp. grated orange zest
- 1 tsp. Ginger
- 1 cup Tea leaves
- 1 cup Brown sugar
- 1 tsp. Cinnamon
- 2 Cloves
- ¼ cup Olive oil
- 3 tbsp. Lemon juice
- The Heat:
- Use charcoal and Applewood chunks for indirect smokes.

- The Water Pan:
- 2 cups orange juice

Directions:

1. Combine Sichuan peppercorns with kosher salt, grated orange zest, ginger, tea leaves, brown sugar, cinnamon, and cloves

2. Pour olive oil and lemon juice over the spice mixture, then stir until incorporated.

3. Rub the quails with the spice mixture and marinate for at least 3 hours. Store in the fridge to keep the quails fresh.

4. Prepare the grill and set it for indirect heat.

5. Place charcoal and starters in a grill, then ignite the starters. Put the burning charcoal on one side of the grill.

6. Place a heavy-duty aluminum pan, then place it on the other side of the grill.

7. Pour orange juice into the aluminum pan, then place wood chunks on top of the burning charcoal. Set the grill grate.

8. Cover the grill with the lid and set the temperature to 200°F (93°C).

9. Place the seasoned quails on the grate inside the grill, then smoke for 2 hours.

10. Once the smoked quails are done, or the smoked quails' internal temperature has reached 160°F (71°C), remove from the grill and transfer to a serving dish.

11. Serve and enjoy.

Nutrition: Amount per 75 g = 1 serving(s) Energy (calories): 175 kcal Protein: 2.12 g Fat: 9.03 g Carbohydrates: 22.45 g

37. Roasted Venison Tenderloin

Preparation Time: 10 minutes

Cooking Time: 28 minutes

Servings: 6

- The Meat:
- 2, each about 1 ½ pound venison tenderloin
- The Marinade:
- ¼ cup dry red wine
- 1 tsp. minced garlic
- 2 tbsp. soy sauce
- 1 tbsp. chopped rosemary
- 1 tsp. ground black pepper
- ½ cup olive oil
- The Seasoning:
- 1 tbsp. salt
- ½ tbsp. ground black pepper
- The Fire:
- According to the user manual, fill the grill's hopper with 2 pounds of wood pellets, apple flavor, and set the grill.
- Switch on the grill, select the "smoke" setting, shut with the lid, and use the control panel to set the temperature to 500 degrees F.

- Wait for 10 to 15 minutes or until the fire starts in the grill and it reaches the set temperature.

Directions:

1. Before preheating the grill, marinate the venison.
2. For this, prepare the marinade; take a small mixing bowl and whisk garlic, wine, and soy sauce until combined.
3. Add black pepper and rosemary, stir until mixed, and then whisk in oil until emulsified.
4. Place venison in a large plastic bag, pour in prepared marinade, seal the bag, turn it upside down to coat venison and let it marinate in the refrigerator for a minimum of 8 hours.
5. Then remove the venison from the marinade, pat dry and then season with salt and black pepper.
6. When the grill has preheated, place venison on the grilling rack, grill for 4 minutes per side until nicely browned, and then continue cooking for 20 minutes until the venison's internal temperature reaches 135 degrees F.
7. When done, let venison rest for 5 minutes, then cut into slices and serve immediately.

Nutrition: Amount per 49 g = 1 serving(s) Energy (calories): 182 kcal Protein: 0.65 g Fat: 19 g

Carbohydrates: 2.63 g

38. Grilled Game Hens with Rosemary sprig

Preparation Time: 20 minutes

Cooking Time: 60minutes

Servings: 4

Ingredients:

The Meat:

- 4 Game hens, giblets removed

The Rub:

- 4 tbsp. melted butter, unsalted
- 4 tsp. chicken rub
- Other Ingredients:
- 4 rosemary sprig
- The Fire:
- According to the user manual, fill the grill's hopper with 2 pounds of wood pellets, any flavor, and set the grill.
- Switch on the grill, select the "smoke" setting, shut with the lid, and use the control panel to set the temperature to 375 degrees F.
- Wait for 10 to 15 minutes or until the fire starts in the grill and it reaches the set temperature.

Directions:

1. In the meantime, prepare hens and for this, rinse well, pat dry, then tuck their wings and tie their legs by using a kitchen string.
2. Then rub melted butter outside of hens, sprinkle with chicken rub, and then place a sprig of rosemary into the cavity of each hen.
3. When the grill has preheated, place hens on the grilling rack and grill for 1 hour or until the control panel shows 165 degrees F's internal temperature, turning halfway.
4. When done, remove hens from the grill and let them rest for 5 minutes.
5. Serve immediately.

Nutrition: Amount per 143 g = 1 serving(s) Energy (calories): 276 kcal Protein: 30.09 g

Fat: 16.66 g Carbohydrates: 0.05 g

39. *Empanadas*

Preparation Time: 20 minutes

Cooking Time: 20 minutes

Servings: 4:

Ingredients:

- 3/4 cup + 1 tbsp all-purpose flour
- ½ tsp baking powder
- 1 tbsp sugar
- ¼ tsp salt or to taste
- 2 tbsp cold water
- 1/3 cups butter
- 1 small egg (beaten)
- Filling:
- ½ small onion (chopped)
- 57g ground beef (1/8 pound)
- 2 tbsp marinara sauce
- 1 small carrot peeled and diced)
- 1/8 small potato (peeled and diced) 35 grams
- 2 tbsp water

- 1 garlic clove (minced)

- 1 tbsp olive oil

- 1 tbsp raisin

- 2 tbsp green peas

- ½ tsp salt or taste

- ½ tsp ground black pepper or to taste

- 1 hard-boiled egg (sliced)

Directions:

1. Start your grill on smoke mode and leave the lid open for 5 minutes, or until the fire starts.

2. Close the grill and preheat the grill to 400°F with the lid closed for 15 minutes, using hickory hardwood pellets.

3. For the fillet, place a cast-iron skillet on the grill and add the oil.

4. Once the oil is hot, add the onion and garlic and sauté until the onion is tender and translucent.

5. Add the ground beef and sauté until it is tender, stirring often.

6. Stir in the marinara, salt, water, and pepper.

7. Bring to a boil and reduce the heat. Cook for 30 seconds.

8. Stir in the carrot, raisin, and potatoes and cook for 3 minutes.

9. Stir in the green peas and sliced egg. Cook for additional 2 minutes, stirring often.

10. Spray a baking dish with a non-stick spray.

11. For the dough, combine the flour, baking powder salt, and sugar in a large mixing bowl. Mix until well combined.

12. Add butter and mix until it is well incorporated.

13. Add egg and mix until you form the dough.

14. Put the dough on a floured surface and knead the dough for a few minutes. Add more flour if the dough is not thick enough.

15. Roll the dough flat with a rolling pin. The flat dough should be ¼ inch thick.

16. Cut the flat dough into circles.

17. Add equal amounts of the beef mixture to the middle of each flat circular dough slice. Fold the dough slice and close the edges by pressing with your fingers or a fork.

18. Arrange the empanadas into the baking sheet in a single layer.

19. Place the baking sheet on the grill and bake for 10 minutes.

20. Remove the baking sheet from the grill and flip the empanadas.

21. Bake for another 10 minutes on the grill or until empanadas is golden brown.

Nutrition: Calories: 353 | Total Fat: 22.3g | Saturated Fat: 11.3g Cholesterol: 129mg | Sodium: 481mg Total Carbohydrate 28.9g Dietary Fiber 1.9g Total Sugars: 6.6g | Protein: 10.4g

CPSIA information can be obtained
at www.ICGtesting.com
Printed in the USA
BVHW040845150621
609626BV00015B/329

9 781914 416941